Montessori for Seniors

Empowering Aging Adults through Independence and Engagement

By Veronica Ricci

Copyright © 2023 Montesenior All rights reserved

The characters and events portrayed in this book are fictitious. Any similarity to real persons, living or dead, is coincidental and not intended by the author.

No part of this book may be reproduced, or stored in a retrieval system, or transmitted in any form or by any means, electronic, mechanical, photocopying, recording, or otherwise, without express written permission of the publisher.

SBN: 9798397416160

Printed in the United States of America

This book is dedicated to my mom Sara Calvo, for all that you taught me... My brother Miguel Torres for being there when I needed you the most... My daughter Giuliana, my whole life, my motivation and my inspiration.

INTRODUCTION 7

SENIOR CARE 11

COMMON CONDITIONS THAT AFFECT SENIORS.. 15

SYMPTOMS OF AGING VS SYMPTOMS OF DEMENTIA 19

THE SENIOR BRAIN AND HOW DECLINE AFFECTS INDEPENDENCE 21

THE MONTESSORI METHOD 25

BENEFITS OF IMPLEMENTING THE MONTESSORI METHOD IN SENIOR LIVING COMMUNITIES 33

CREATING THE PREPARED ENVIRONMENT 37

PROMOTING INDEPENDENCE AND AUTONOMY . 43

INDIVIDUALIZED LEARNING AND ENGAGEMENT . 47

COGNITIVE STIMULATION AND MEMORY SUPPORT 53

STAFF TRAINING AND IMPLEMENTATION 57

REAL LIFE EXAMPLES OF SUCCESSFUL IMPLEMENTATION OF MONTESSORI FOR SENIORS 61

INTRODUCTION

As the world's population continues to age, it becomes increasingly important to focus on promoting active aging and maintaining independence among seniors. Active aging refers to the process of optimizing opportunities for health, participation, and security in order to enhance the quality of life as people age. It involves physical, mental, and social engagement that allows seniors to lead fulfilling and meaningful lives.

Physical Health and Well-being:
- a. Regular physical activity: Engaging in regular exercise and physical activity is crucial for seniors to maintain their physical health, strength, and mobility. It helps prevent chronic diseases, reduces the risk of falls, and improves overall well-being.
- b. Enhancing longevity: Active aging promotes longevity by reducing the risk of age-related illnesses and maintaining a healthy body weight. It enables seniors to live independently and enjoy a higher quality of life in their later years.

Cognitive Function:
- a. Mental stimulation: Staying mentally active through lifelong learning, engaging in cognitive activities, and pursuing hobbies helps maintain cognitive function and prevent cognitive decline.

Active aging promotes brain health and can reduce the risk of developing conditions such as dementia and Alzheimer's disease.
- b. Memory retention and cognitive abilities: Engaging in intellectually stimulating activities, such as reading, puzzles, and social interactions, helps seniors retain their memory and cognitive abilities. It allows them to remain mentally sharp and actively participate in daily life.

Social Engagement:
- a. Emotional well-being: Active aging encourages social interactions, which play a vital role in seniors' emotional well-being. Staying connected with family, friends, and the community helps combat loneliness, depression, and anxiety.
- b. Sense of purpose and belonging: Maintaining an active social life provides seniors with a sense of purpose and belonging. Participating in social activities, volunteer work, or joining clubs and organizations fosters a sense of community, strengthens social networks, and promotes overall life satisfaction.

Independence and Autonomy:
- a. Personal empowerment: Active aging empowers seniors by enabling them to retain control over their lives. It allows them to make choices, engage in activities of their choice, and maintain a sense of autonomy.

- b. Reducing dependence: By actively engaging in physical, mental, and social activities, seniors can reduce their reliance on others for daily tasks and support. This independence enhances their self-esteem, confidence, and overall quality of life.

Active aging and maintaining independence are essential for seniors to lead fulfilling and meaningful lives. By promoting physical health, cognitive function, social engagement, and independence, we can support seniors in maximizing their well-being and quality of life. Governments, communities, and individuals must recognize the significance of active aging and create opportunities and environments that enable seniors to age actively and independently. Embracing active aging not only benefits seniors but also contributes to the overall well-being of society as a whole.

Chapter 1

SENIOR CARE

Senior care is a crucial aspect of our society, as the elderly population continues to grow. It is important to ensure that our seniors receive the care and attention they need to live a comfortable and fulfilling life. There are various types of senior care available, including in-home care, assisted living facilities, and nursing homes.

In-home care is a popular option for seniors who wish to remain in their own homes. This type of care involves a caregiver coming to the senior's home to provide assistance with daily tasks such as bathing, dressing, and meal preparation. In-home care can also include companionship and transportation to appointments.

Assisted living facilities are another option for seniors who require more assistance with daily tasks but do not require the level of medical care provided in a nursing home. These facilities provide a range of services, including meals, housekeeping, and assistance with medication management.

Nursing homes are designed for seniors who require around-the-clock medical care and supervision. These facilities provide skilled nursing care, rehabilitation services, and assistance with daily tasks.

Regardless of the type of senior care chosen, it is important to ensure that the facility or caregiver is reputable and provides quality care. Seniors deserve to be treated with respect and dignity, and it is our responsibility as a society to ensure that they receive the care they need and deserve.

Here are some tips for senior care:

1. Establish a routine: People with dementia thrive on routine and familiarity. Establishing a daily routine can help them feel more secure and reduce anxiety.

2. Simplify the environment: Simplify the environment by removing clutter and unnecessary items. This can help reduce confusion and agitation.

3. Use visual cues: Use visual cues such as signs and labels to help seniors with dementia navigate their environment.

4. Provide meaningful activities: Engage seniors with dementia in meaningful activities such as music, art, and reminiscing. This can help improve their mood and cognitive function.

5. Be patient and compassionate: Seniors with dementia may become confused, agitated, or upset. It's important to be patient and compassionate, and to avoid arguing or correcting them.

6. Ensure safety: Ensure that the senior's environment is safe and secure. This may involve installing safety features such as grab bars and handrails, or using monitoring devices.

7. Seek support: Caring for a senior with dementia can be challenging. Seek support from family, friends, or a professional caregiver to help manage the responsibilities and reduce stress.

Montessori classes/activities have been proven to be beneficial when caring for seniors and is very important to understand the Montessori method is more than just materials and education, is a philosophy based on respect, kindness and making sure there's a prepared environment that provides what the individual needs. By using this method with seniors we can help prevent and ease many symptoms of aging.

Chapter 2

COMMON CONDITIONS THAT AFFECT SENIORS

There are several common conditions that affect seniors, including:

1. Arthritis: This is a condition that causes inflammation and pain in the joints.

2. Osteoporosis: This is a condition that causes bones to become weak and brittle, increasing the risk of fractures.

3. Alzheimer's disease and other forms of dementia: These are conditions that affect memory, thinking, and behavior.

4. Cardiovascular disease: This includes conditions such as heart disease, stroke, and high blood pressure.

5. Diabetes: This is a condition that affects the body's ability to regulate blood sugar levels.

6. Respiratory diseases: These include conditions such as chronic obstructive pulmonary disease (COPD) and asthma.

7. Cancer: Seniors are at an increased risk of developing cancer, particularly breast, prostate, and lung cancer.

8. Depression: This is a common condition among seniors, often related to social isolation, loss of loved ones, and other life changes.

9. Vision and hearing loss: These are common age-related conditions that can affect quality of life and independence.

10. Falls: Seniors are at an increased risk of falls, which can lead to serious injuries and complications.

As people age, they may experience a variety of symptoms and pains. Some common symptoms and pains that seniors may experience include:

1. Joint pain and stiffness: This is a common symptom of arthritis, which affects many seniors.

2. Fatigue: Seniors may experience fatigue due to a variety of factors, including medication side effects, chronic health conditions, and sleep disturbances.

3. Memory problems: Many seniors experience some degree of memory loss as they age, which can be a normal

part of the aging process or a symptom of a more serious condition like dementia.

4. Vision and hearing problems: Seniors may experience changes in their vision and hearing as they age, which can impact their quality of life.

5. Digestive issues: Seniors may experience digestive issues like constipation, diarrhea, and acid reflux.

6. Breathing difficulties: Seniors may experience breathing difficulties due to chronic obstructive pulmonary disease (COPD), asthma, or other respiratory conditions.

7. Skin changes: Seniors may experience changes in their skin, including dryness, thinning, and age spots.

Chapter 3

SYMPTOMS OF AGING VS SYMPTOMS OF DEMENTIA

As we age, our bodies and minds undergo various changes. Some of these changes are a natural part of the aging process, while others may be indicative of a more serious condition, such as dementia. While both aging and dementia can cause similar symptoms, there are some key differences between the two.

Aging is a natural process that affects everyone. As we age, our bodies undergo various changes, such as a decrease in muscle mass, a decrease in bone density, and a decrease in cognitive function. These changes can lead to a variety of symptoms, such as fatigue, weakness, and forgetfulness. However, these symptoms are generally mild and do not significantly impact our daily lives.

Dementia, on the other hand, is a progressive condition that affects the brain. It is characterized by a decline in cognitive function, including memory loss, difficulty with language, and impaired judgment. Dementia can also cause changes in mood and behavior, such as depression, anxiety, and aggression. Unlike the mild symptoms of aging, the symptoms of dementia are often severe and can significantly impact a person's ability to function independently.

One of the key differences between the symptoms of aging and dementia is the severity of the symptoms. While aging can cause mild symptoms that do not significantly impact our daily lives, dementia can cause severe symptoms that can make it difficult to perform even the most basic tasks. Additionally, the symptoms of dementia tend to get worse over time, while the symptoms of aging generally remain stable.

Another difference between the symptoms of aging and dementia is the age at which they occur. While aging is a natural process that occurs over time, dementia is a condition that can affect people of all ages, including children.

In conclusion, while aging and dementia can cause similar symptoms, there are some key differences between the two. Aging is a natural process that affects everyone and can cause mild symptoms that do not significantly impact our daily lives. Dementia, on the other hand, is a progressive condition that affects the brain and can cause severe symptoms that can make it difficult to function independently. Understanding the differences between these two conditions can help us better identify and manage the symptoms.

Chapter 4

THE SENIOR BRAIN AND HOW DECLINE AFFECTS INDEPENDENCE

Aging affects our brain function. Unfortunately, these changes can lead to a decline in cognitive abilities, which can have a significant impact on our daily lives.

One of the most significant changes that occur in the brain is a decrease in the number of neurons, the cells in the brain that are responsible for transmitting information. This decline can manifest in a variety of ways, including difficulty with memory, attention, and problem-solving.

Another factor that contributes to the decline in brain function with aging is a decrease in the production of neurotransmitters. Neurotransmitters are chemicals in the brain that are responsible for transmitting signals between neurons. This decline can manifest in a variety of ways, including difficulty with mood regulation, sleep, and appetite.

In addition to these changes, aging can also lead to a decline in the brain's ability to form new connections between neurons. This decline can make it more difficult for the brain to adapt to new situations and learn new information. This can lead to a decline in cognitive abilities, including difficulty with memory and problem-solving.

Finally, aging can also lead to an increase in inflammation in the brain. Inflammation is the body's response to injury or infection, and it can have a negative impact on brain function. Inflammation in the brain can also affect memory, attention, and problem-solving.

Brain function declines with aging due to a variety of factors, while these changes are a natural part of the aging process, there are steps that individuals can take to help maintain their cognitive abilities, including engaging in regular exercise, eating a healthy diet, and engaging in mentally stimulating activities.

One of the most significant ways that brain decline can affect independence is through the loss of memory. As we age, our ability to remember things can become impaired, making it difficult to perform everyday tasks such as remembering appointments, taking medication, or even finding our way around our own home. This can lead to a loss of independence as we become more reliant on others to help us with these tasks.

Also, our ability to make decisions can become impaired, making it difficult to manage our finances, make important medical decisions, or even decide what to eat for dinner.

In addition to memory and decision-making, brain decline can also affect our physical abilities. Our motor skills change, making it difficult to perform everyday tasks such as cooking, cleaning, or even getting dressed.
So, what can be done to mitigate the effects of brain decline on independence? One solution is to engage in activities that promote brain health, such as exercise, socializing, and learning new things. These activities can help to keep the brain active and healthy, which can slow down the decline in cognitive function.

Brain decline can have a significant impact on our ability to maintain independence as we age. However, by engaging in activities that promote brain health and seeking out assistance when needed, individuals can mitigate the effects of brain decline and maintain their independence for as long as possible.

Chapter 5

THE MONTESSORI METHOD

Maria Montessori, an Italian physician and educator, is widely recognized for her revolutionary approach to education. Born in 1870, Montessori was a pioneer in the field of child development and her educational philosophy continues to have a profound impact on education systems worldwide. Montessori's approach is rooted in her belief that children are naturally eager learners and that they possess an innate curiosity and drive for exploration. Her work, however, extends beyond the realm of early childhood education and has also been adapted for other age groups, including seniors.

Montessori's philosophy is based on several key principles that form the foundation of her educational approach. These principles include independence, self-directed learning, and respect for individuality.

A. Independence: A fundamental principle of the Montessori philosophy is the promotion of independence in learners. Montessori recognized that fostering independence in children and adults alike is crucial for their development and growth. In her educational approach, she created an environment that encouraged learners to actively engage with their surroundings and take responsibility for their own learning. By providing age-appropriate materials and tools, Montessori aimed to empower individuals to perform tasks independently and develop a sense of self-reliance.

B.   Self-directed Learning: Montessori believed that individuals have an innate drive for learning and that they learn best when they can follow their own interests and passions. In her approach, she emphasized self-directed learning, which allows learners to choose their activities and work at their own pace. Montessori classrooms, for example, are carefully prepared environments that provide a wide range of materials and activities, allowing learners to explore and learn based on their individual preferences and curiosities. This approach fosters a love for learning and encourages intrinsic motivation in learners.

C.   Respect for Individuality: Respect for the individuality of each learner is a core principle of Montessori philosophy. Montessori recognized that every person is unique and has their own set of strengths, interests, and learning styles. Therefore, her approach emphasizes tailoring education to meet the needs of each individual learner. Montessori classrooms promote individualized instruction, allowing learners to progress at their own pace and engage with materials that suit their specific developmental stage and interests. This approach respects the diverse abilities and learning preferences of individuals and nurtures a sense of self-worth and belonging.

By incorporating these key principles into her educational approach, Maria Montessori revolutionized traditional teaching methods and created an environment that empowers learners to become active participants in their own education. Her emphasis on independence, self-directed learning, and respect for individuality has inspired educators worldwide to rethink traditional approaches to education and to create learning environments that foster autonomy, curiosity, and a lifelong love for learning.

Furthermore, the Montessori principles have also found application beyond early childhood education, with adaptations for other age groups. The principles of independence, self-directed learning, and respect for individuality remain relevant and beneficial in promoting engagement, well-being, and a sense of purpose among seniors. By embracing these principles, Montessori for seniors can empower aging adults and enhance their quality of life in various senior care settings.

The Montessori approach has found a meaningful application in senior care settings through the adaptation of its principles. As aging adults face unique challenges and changes in physical, cognitive, and emotional well-being, the Montessori philosophy offers a valuable framework to support their needs. By adapting Montessori principles for seniors, we can create environments that promote independence, engagement, and a sense of purpose, ultimately enhancing their quality of life.

One of the key principles of the Montessori philosophy, independence, remains relevant and significant for seniors. As individuals age, maintaining a sense of autonomy and self-reliance becomes increasingly important. Adaptations can be made by designing senior living spaces that are accessible and supportive of independent functioning. This may include incorporating grab bars, adjustable furniture, and accessible tools that enable seniors to perform daily tasks with ease and confidence. Empowering seniors to make choices and decisions regarding their care, activities, and daily routines further enhances their independence and self-esteem.

Another principle, self-directed learning, can be adapted to facilitate continued growth and cognitive stimulation for seniors. Engaging seniors in purposeful and meaningful activities that align with their interests and abilities promotes a sense of accomplishment and fulfillment. By providing a range of options for seniors to explore, such as creative arts, music, gardening, or lifelong learning opportunities, we support their ongoing intellectual development and encourage a love for learning. Seniors can take the lead in determining the pace and depth of their engagement, fostering a sense of autonomy and curiosity.

Respect for individuality is a crucial aspect of the Montessori philosophy and its adaptation for seniors. Each senior has a unique life history, preferences, and abilities. By recognizing and honoring their individuality, caregivers and senior living communities can create person-centered care plans and personalized activities that cater to their specific needs and interests. This individualized approach promotes a sense of value, dignity, and belonging, fostering emotional well-being and a positive self-image among seniors.

Successful aging is a multidimensional concept that encompasses physical, cognitive, and psychosocial well-being. The principles of the Montessori philosophy align closely with the goals of successful aging, making it a natural fit for senior care. The adaptation of Montessori principles for seniors can contribute to their overall well-being and enhance their journey of successful aging. Promoting independence among seniors is a key factor in successful aging. The Montessori approach emphasizes the importance of supporting seniors in maintaining their independence and self-reliance. By creating environments that enable independent functioning and empowering seniors to actively participate in their care and daily activities, we promote their physical and emotional well-being. This, in turn, contributes to their overall sense of fulfillment and successful aging.

Engagement and purpose are also essential components of successful aging, and the Montessori approach offers effective strategies to foster both. By providing seniors with meaningful activities and opportunities to contribute to their community, we promote a sense of purpose and belonging. Engagement in purposeful tasks stimulates cognitive functioning, enhances physical well-being, and cultivates social connections. The Montessori principles of self-directed learning and individualized care allow seniors to pursue activities that align with their interests and abilities, creating a sense of purpose and joy in their everyday lives.

Additionally, the Montessori philosophy recognizes the importance of social interaction and collaboration. Seniors thrive in environments that foster meaningful relationships and provide opportunities for social engagement. By designing community spaces and activities that encourage peer interaction, collaboration, and shared experiences, we enhance social connectedness, emotional well-being, and successful aging.

Adapting Montessori principles for seniors presents a promising approach to senior care that aligns with the goals of successful aging. By promoting independence, self-directed learning, and respect for individuality, we create environments that empower seniors, support their cognitive and emotional well-being, and foster a sense of purpose and engagement. The Montessori philosophy offers a transformative framework that can enhance the quality of life for seniors, enabling them to age gracefully and successfully.

Chapter 6

BENEFITS OF IMPLEMENTING THE MONTESSORI METHOD IN SENIOR LIVING COMMUNITIES

Implementing the Montessori approach in senior living communities offers several benefits for aging adults.

Some of the key benefits include:

- Independence and Autonomy: The Montessori approach promotes independence and autonomy by encouraging seniors to actively engage in self-directed activities and make choices based on their preferences and abilities.

- Engagement and Purpose: By providing meaningful activities and opportunities for learning, the Montessori approach keeps seniors engaged and helps them maintain a sense of purpose, fostering their overall well-being and quality of life.

- Cognitive Stimulation: The Montessori method incorporates cognitive stimulation through various activities, games, and exercises, which can help improve cognitive functioning, memory, and problem-solving skills in seniors.

- Social Interaction: Montessori-based senior living communities create an environment that encourages social interaction and collaboration among residents, fostering a sense of community and reducing feelings of loneliness or isolation.

- Individualized Care: The Montessori approach recognizes the unique abilities, interests, and needs of each senior. By providing individualized care and tailoring activities to their specific capabilities, it supports personalized and person-centered care.

- Dignity and Respect: The Montessori philosophy emphasizes treating each individual with dignity and respect, honoring their autonomy and choices, and promoting a positive self-image among seniors.

- Empowerment and Self-Esteem: Through engaging in purposeful activities and experiencing success, seniors in Montessori-based communities can enhance their self-esteem, confidence, and feelings of empowerment.

- Mental and Physical Well-being: The Montessori approach focuses on promoting holistic well-being. By offering a range of activities that stimulate mental, physical, and emotional health, it contributes to overall wellness and can even help reduce the risk of cognitive decline and physical deterioration.

- Reminiscence and Life Review: Incorporating reminiscence therapy and life review techniques, Montessori-based programs help seniors connect with their past, reminisce about meaningful experiences, and share their life stories with others.

- Staff and Caregiver Satisfaction: Implementing the Montessori approach in senior living communities can also lead to increased staff and caregiver satisfaction. The approach offers a more person-centered and fulfilling approach to care, enhancing job satisfaction and creating a positive work environment.

It's important to note that the benefits may vary based on individual needs and the specific implementation of the Montessori approach in each senior living community.

Chapter 7
CREATING THE PREPARED ENVIRONMENT

1. Importance of the Physical Environment in Supporting Seniors' Independence

The physical environment plays a crucial role in senior care settings, as it can greatly impact the well-being and independence of aging adults. Designing an enriching environment that promotes independence aligns with the core principles of the Montessori philosophy.

1.1 Enhancing Autonomy and Mobility:
A well-designed physical environment empowers seniors to navigate their surroundings independently. By incorporating features such as handrails, non-slip flooring, and clear pathways, mobility is facilitated, reducing the risk of falls and promoting a sense of confidence. Accessibility features, such as ramps or elevators, should be considered to enable easy movement between floors and areas.

1.2 Promoting Safety and Comfort:
Creating a safe and comfortable environment is paramount for seniors. Adequate lighting, including natural light

sources, reduces the risk of accidents and improves mood. Proper temperature control and ventilation ensure a comfortable living space. Moreover, minimizing noise levels and incorporating comfortable seating areas provide a peaceful and relaxing ambiance, enhancing overall well-being.

---

2. Designing a Senior-Friendly Environment Based on Montessori Principles

2.1 The Prepared Environment:
The Montessori approach emphasizes the concept of a prepared environment, tailored to meet the needs and abilities of seniors. Design spaces that allow for independence and engagement, offering choices that align with their preferences and capabilities. Ensure that the environment is organized, clutter-free, and visually appealing, promoting a sense of order and calmness.

2.2 Accessible and Age-Appropriate Materials:
Provide seniors with age-appropriate materials and tools that support their independence. Consider adaptive devices and equipment that enable individuals with physical limitations to engage in activities without assistance. Ensure that materials are easily accessible and arranged in a manner that encourages exploration and self-directed learning.

3. Incorporating Sensory Stimulation and Accessibility in the Environment

3.1 Sensory Stimulation:
Incorporating sensory stimulation into the environment is essential for seniors' cognitive and emotional well-being. Engage different senses by introducing textures, colors, and scents in the environment. Consider incorporating sensory gardens, where seniors can experience the therapeutic benefits of nature through touch, smell, and sight.

3.2 Accessible and Engaging Activities:
Design spaces that facilitate a variety of engaging activities for seniors. Consider activity stations where individuals can participate in hobbies, puzzles, or creative endeavors. These areas should be accessible and well-equipped, allowing seniors to pursue their interests independently. Incorporate elements such as art supplies, reading materials, or musical instruments to provide diverse engagement opportunities.

4. Organizing Spaces for Easy Navigation and Engagement

4.1 Clear Signage and Visual Cues:
Seniors may face challenges with navigation and orientation. Implement clear signage and visual cues throughout the environment, including large and readable signs, color-coded areas, and pictures/icons that help individuals locate different spaces and facilities independently.

4.2 Intuitive Layout and Design:
Organize spaces with a logical layout that facilitates easy navigation. Consider creating clearly defined areas for different activities, such as dining, socializing, and relaxation. Arrange furniture and equipment in a manner that allows for easy movement and encourages interaction with others.

5. Using Natural Materials and Incorporating Elements of Nature

5.1 Biophilic Design:
Integrating elements of nature into the environment can have a profound impact on seniors' well-being. Incorporate natural materials such as wood, plants, and water features to create a calming and rejuvenating atmosphere. Provide access to outdoor spaces, such as gardens or courtyards, where seniors can enjoy fresh air, sunshine, and connect with nature.

5.2 Sensory Gardens and Outdoor Spaces:
Design sensory gardens that engage seniors' senses through the use of scented flowers, textured plants, and soothing sounds of nature. Create outdoor spaces that offer seating, walking paths, and opportunities for gentle exercise, promoting physical activity and a sense of connection with the natural world.

The physical environment in senior care settings has a significant impact on their independence, well-being, and overall quality of life. By designing a senior-friendly environment based on Montessori principles, we can promote autonomy, engage the senses, and create a nurturing space that supports seniors' physical, cognitive, and emotional needs. Incorporating sensory stimulation, ensuring accessibility, and incorporating elements of nature are key considerations in creating an enriching environment that fosters independence and enhances seniors' overall experience in their living community.

Chapter 8

PROMOTING INDEPENDENCE AND AUTONOMY

Promoting independence and autonomy among seniors is essential for their overall well-being and quality of life. The following are some strategies for increasing autonomy in senior care:

- Personal Care and Daily Living Skills:
Encourage seniors to engage in activities that promote self-care and independence, such as dressing, grooming, and meal preparation. Provide adaptive tools and techniques, as necessary, to support their abilities and make these tasks more manageable. Encourage them to perform these activities at their own pace, fostering a sense of accomplishment and self-reliance.

- Self-Monitoring and Health Management:
Support seniors in taking an active role in managing their health. Help them develop routines for medication management, encourage them to track their health indicators, and provide education on self-monitoring techniques. By empowering seniors to be involved in their

own healthcare, they gain a sense of control and responsibility, promoting their independence.

- Activity Options and Variety:

Offer a wide range of activities that cater to different interests and abilities. Provide choices in recreational activities, hobbies, and social engagements. Seniors should have the freedom to choose activities that align with their preferences, enabling them to explore new interests and engage in activities that bring them joy and fulfillment.

- Individualized Activity Plans:

Develop individualized activity plans that consider each senior's unique needs and preferences. Collaborate with seniors to identify their interests and goals, and incorporate those into their activity plans. By involving seniors in decision-making and tailoring activities to their individual needs, you promote a sense of ownership and autonomy.

- Assistive Devices and Technology:

Introduce assistive devices and technology to support seniors with cognitive or physical limitations. These can include adaptive tools for eating, dressing, or mobility aids such as walkers or wheelchairs. Assistive technology, such as voice-activated devices or memory aids, can also enhance independence and engagement for seniors with cognitive challenges.

- Task Simplification and Sequencing:

Break down complex tasks into manageable steps and provide visual cues or written instructions to aid in comprehension and execution. Simplifying tasks helps seniors with cognitive impairments or memory loss maintain independence by reducing confusion and frustration. Focus on maintaining their engagement and providing appropriate support throughout the task.

- Shared Responsibilities and Collaborative Decision-Making:

Involve seniors in decision-making regarding daily tasks and routines. Encourage their participation in planning and organizing activities such as meal preparation, household chores, or community events. By actively involving seniors in these processes, they feel a sense of purpose and contribution to the community.

- Empowering Seniors in Personal Spaces:

Support seniors in maintaining their personal spaces, such as their living quarters. Encourage them to decorate their space, arrange furniture, and personalize it according to their tastes and preferences. This autonomy in personal spaces fosters a sense of identity, control, and comfort.

- Meaningful Engagement and Purposeful Activities:

Offer opportunities for seniors to engage in activities that provide a sense of purpose and accomplishment. This can include volunteering, mentoring, or participating in creative projects. By promoting meaningful engagement, seniors maintain a sense of identity, contribute to the community, and experience a sense of fulfillment.

- Celebrating Achievements and Milestones:

Recognize and celebrate seniors' achievements and milestones, regardless of their size. This can involve acknowledging personal accomplishments, birthdays, or other special occasions. By acknowledging and celebrating these moments, seniors are reminded of their value and worth, promoting their self-esteem and a positive outlook.

By fostering self-care skills, encouraging decision-making and choice, providing adaptive strategies, facilitating active participation, and supporting a sense of purpose and accomplishment, we empower seniors to maintain their independence, enhance their self-esteem, and experience a greater sense of satisfaction and fulfillment in their daily lives. By incorporating Montessori principles, we create an environment that respects and nurtures their autonomy, promoting a positive aging experience.

Chapter 9

INDIVIDUALIZED LEARNING AND ENGAGEMENT

Unlocking the Potencial of Seniors

In the realm of senior care and education, recognizing the uniqueness of each individual is crucial to fostering meaningful engagement and promoting lifelong learning. Individualized learning and engagement approaches allow seniors to pursue activities that align with their abilities, interests, and preferences, leading to enhanced well-being and a sense of fulfillment.

Seniors, like people of any age, possess a wide range of abilities and interests. Recognizing and appreciating these individual qualities is the first step in designing effective learning and engagement experiences. By conducting assessments and establishing rapport, caregivers and educators can gain insights into seniors' strengths, weaknesses, and personal preferences. Understanding their abilities and interests allows for the creation of tailored approaches that cater to their unique needs, ensuring a more fulfilling learning experience.

To promote engagement and maximize learning outcomes, activities and learning experiences must be tailored to individual needs. This customization involves adapting materials, instructions, and pacing to match seniors' cognitive and physical abilities. Modifying activities not only ensures that seniors can actively participate but also enhances their self-confidence and motivation. By personalizing learning experiences, seniors are more likely to achieve success, leading to a deeper sense of satisfaction and a desire for continued learning.

Offering a diverse range of activities is essential for promoting engagement among seniors. By providing mental, physical, and social activities, caregivers and educators cater to the holistic well-being of seniors. Mental engagement can be fostered through puzzles, memory games, or brain exercises that challenge cognitive abilities. Physical activities, such as exercise programs or sensory stimulation, promote physical well-being and maintain mobility. Social activities, including group discussions or social events, encourage interpersonal connections and combat social isolation. The variety of activities ensures that seniors have opportunities to engage in areas they enjoy, fostering a sense of purpose and satisfaction.

Peer interaction and collaboration are key components of a comprehensive learning experience for seniors. By creating opportunities for seniors to interact with their peers, caregivers and educators foster a sense of community and connection. Group activities, clubs, and shared interest groups provide spaces where seniors can learn from one another, share experiences, and build friendships. Collaboration in problem-solving activities encourages teamwork and promotes a sense of achievement. Peer interaction not only enhances social engagement but also provides a platform for emotional support and growth.

Individualized learning and engagement approaches have the power to unlock the potential of seniors by recognizing their uniqueness, tailoring activities to their needs, offering a diverse range of engagement opportunities, and encouraging peer interaction and collaboration. By personalizing learning experiences, seniors are empowered to actively participate in activities that align with their abilities, interests, and preferences. This approach promotes overall well-being, stimulates cognitive and physical functioning, and fosters a sense of belonging. As we embrace individualization in senior education and care, we honor the value and potential of each senior, enabling them to thrive in their pursuit of lifelong learning and engagement.

Incorporating Reminiscence Therapy and Life Review Techniques

Reminiscence therapy involves the process of recalling and reflecting on past experiences, while life review techniques delve deeper into the examination of one's life as a whole. Both approaches tap into the power of memories and personal stories to improve seniors' mental, emotional, and social well-being. Benefits of Reminiscence Therapy include:

- Enhancing Emotional Well-being: Engaging in reminiscence therapy and life review can evoke positive emotions, such as joy, happiness, and a sense of accomplishment. By revisiting meaningful moments from the past, seniors experience emotional validation, increased self-esteem, and a renewed sense of purpose.

- Promoting Cognitive Functioning: Recalling memories and engaging in reflective exercises stimulates cognitive functioning. These therapies improve attention, concentration, and memory recall, helping to maintain cognitive abilities and potentially slowing cognitive decline.

- Fostering Communication and Relationships: Reminiscing about the past encourages social interaction and connection. Seniors can share stories with their peers, family members, and caregivers, leading to improved communication, empathy, and understanding. This sharing of personal narratives builds stronger relationships and a sense of community within senior care settings.

Methods of Implementation:

- Storytelling and Conversation: Encourage seniors to share their stories and memories through one-on-one conversations or group settings. Providing a supportive and non-judgmental environment allows seniors to express themselves freely and fosters meaningful connections among participants.

- Memory-Triggering Materials: Utilize visual aids, such as photographs, music, or familiar objects, to stimulate memory recall. These prompts can evoke memories and emotions, facilitating conversations and reminiscence sessions.

- Life Review Exercises: Guide seniors through structured life review exercises that prompt reflection on different aspects of their lives, such as significant relationships, accomplishments, or life lessons. This structured approach aids in deeper self-reflection and a greater sense of self-awareness.

- Multi-Sensory Approaches: Engage multiple senses to enhance the reminiscence experience. Utilize music, scents, or tactile objects associated with specific memories to stimulate a more vivid recollection of past experiences.

Incorporating reminiscence therapy and life review techniques can have a profound impact on seniors' well-being. It promotes a positive self-image, reduces feelings of loneliness or isolation, and provides an opportunity for emotional expression. Seniors gain a renewed sense of purpose, as their memories and experiences are validated and cherished. These therapies strengthen social connections, fostering a sense of belonging and community among seniors.

Chapter 10

COGNITIVE STIMULATION AND MEMORY SUPPORT

Cognitive stimulation and memory support are vital components of senior care, particularly for individuals facing cognitive decline or memory challenges. This chapter explores strategies for enhancing cognitive functioning, implementing memory games and exercises, creating memory-friendly environments and routines, utilizing Montessori-based tools for memory support, and supporting seniors with dementia and cognitive impairments.

Strategies for Enhancing Cognitive Functioning in Seniors:

1. Mental Stimulation: Encourage seniors to engage in mentally stimulating activities such as reading, puzzles, or learning new skills. These activities promote neural connections, improve memory, and enhance cognitive functioning.

2. Physical Exercise: Regular physical exercise has been linked to improved cognitive function and memory retention. Encourage seniors to participate in activities such as walking, yoga, or tai chi, which promote blood flow to the brain and support cognitive health.

3. Social Interaction: Encourage seniors to maintain social connections, as social engagement stimulates cognitive functioning. Group activities, conversations, and community involvement provide opportunities for mental stimulation and promote memory support.

Implementing Memory Games, Puzzles, and Brain Exercises:

- Memory Games: Incorporate memory games that challenge seniors' recall abilities, such as matching games, word association, or trivia quizzes. These games engage memory processes, improve cognitive flexibility, and promote mental acuity.

- Puzzles: Offer a variety of puzzles, such as jigsaw puzzles, Sudoku, or crossword puzzles, to stimulate problem-solving skills and memory recall. These activities promote cognitive engagement and can be adapted to different ability levels.

- Brain Exercises: Introduce brain exercises specifically designed to enhance cognitive functioning, such as memory exercises, attention-training tasks, or cognitive training programs available through digital platforms or apps.

Creating a Memory-Friendly Environment and Routines:

- Organization and Structure: Establish an organized and structured environment to support memory function. Use labels, signs, or visual cues to assist with navigation and finding items. Clearly define spaces and incorporate consistent routines to provide a sense of familiarity and ease cognitive load.

- Memory Aids and Reminders: Provide memory aids, such as calendars, whiteboards, or digital devices, to help seniors remember appointments, tasks, and important information. These aids serve as external memory supports and reduce reliance on internal memory recall.

Using Montessori-Based Tools for Memory Support:

- Memory Boxes or Memory Books: Create memory boxes or books that contain meaningful items or photographs from seniors' pasts. These Montessori-based tools facilitate reminiscence, evoke memories, and promote cognitive stimulation.

- Montessori Activity Trays: Utilize Montessori activity trays that incorporate sensory materials, objects, or sorting tasks to engage cognitive processes and support memory retrieval. These trays can be customized to match seniors' interests and abilities.

Supporting Seniors with Dementia and Cognitive Impairments:

- Person-Centered Care: Adopt a person-centered approach that focuses on understanding the unique needs, abilities, and preferences of seniors with dementia or cognitive impairments. Tailor activities and interventions to support their cognitive function and provide opportunities for engagement.

- Validation and Reminiscence Therapy: Implement validation techniques and reminiscence therapy to support memory and emotional well-being in individuals with dementia. These approaches honor their personal experiences, validate their emotions, and promote a sense of identity and connection.

Implementing strategies for enhancing cognitive functioning, incorporating memory games and exercises, creating memory-friendly environments and routines, and providing support for seniors with dementia and cognitive impairments, caregivers can foster cognitive engagement, promote memory retention, and enhance the overall well-being of seniors.

Chapter 11

STAFF TRAINING AND IMPLEMENTATION

Staff training plays a pivotal role in implementing Montessori principles and practices effectively in senior care settings. Educating caregivers on the philosophy and benefits of Montessori for seniors, providing practical guidance for incorporating Montessori into daily care routines, overcoming challenges, and continuously assessing and improving the Montessori program are all essential components of staff training.

To successfully implement Montessori principles in senior care, it is crucial to provide caregivers with a comprehensive understanding of the philosophy and benefits of Montessori for seniors. Caregivers need to grasp the principles of independence, self-directed learning, and respect for individuality and understand how these principles can enhance the well-being and quality of life of seniors. By imparting this knowledge, caregivers gain insights into the unique needs of seniors and can adapt their approach to provide more person-centered care.

Training caregivers in practical strategies for incorporating Montessori principles into daily care routines equips them with the necessary skills to create an environment that fosters independence and engagement. Caregivers can learn techniques for promoting autonomy, such as providing choices and creating personalized care plans. They can also learn to design activities and learning experiences that cater to seniors' individual interests and abilities. Practical guidance empowers caregivers to implement Montessori principles effectively, ensuring that seniors receive personalized and meaningful care.

Training equips caregivers with tools to overcome challenges that may arise in senior care settings. Caregivers learn to adapt the Montessori approach to different care settings, such as assisted living facilities, memory care units, or in-home care. They gain the ability to address cognitive or physical limitations of seniors, making necessary adjustments to activities or modifying the environment. Training ensures that caregivers are prepared to provide tailored care to meet the diverse needs of seniors.

Staff training is not a one-time event but an ongoing process. It involves continuous assessment and improvement of the Montessori program. Caregivers need to understand the importance of monitoring the effectiveness of their implementation of Montessori principles and practices. Regular assessment allows caregivers to identify areas for improvement and make necessary adjustments to better meet the needs of seniors.

Ongoing training and professional development opportunities enable caregivers to stay up-to-date with new research and best practices in Montessori-based senior care.

By equipping caregivers with the necessary knowledge, skills, and tools, staff training ensures that seniors receive personalized, engaging, and empowering care rooted in the principles of Montessori philosophy.

Chapter 12

REAL LIFE EXAMPLES OF SUCCESSFUL IMPLEMENTATION OF MONTESSORI FOR SENIORS

The Montessori approach has shown remarkable potential in transforming the lives of seniors, enhancing their well-being, and improving their overall quality of life. This chapter shares inspiring real-life examples of successful implementation of Montessori for seniors, highlighting the positive outcomes and demonstrating the impact of the Montessori approach on seniors' well-being. These stories serve as a source of inspiration for caregivers and senior care professionals, reinforcing the value of the Montessori philosophy in senior care.

John's Journey to Independence:

John, a senior living with cognitive impairments, had struggled with feelings of frustration and dependence. Through the implementation of Montessori principles, his caregivers provided him with adaptive tools and activities that matched his interests and abilities. They created a personalized memory box filled with meaningful items from his past, allowing him to reminisce and engage in purposeful conversations. Over time, John's confidence grew, and he developed new skills. He became more independent in his daily activities and experienced a sense of accomplishment and joy. His transformation inspired both his caregivers and fellow residents, showcasing the power of the Montessori approach in promoting independence and enhancing well-being.

Maria's Rediscovered Passion:

Maria, an elderly woman living in a senior community, had always been passionate about art but had lost touch with her creative side over the years. With the implementation of Montessori-based activities, her caregivers recognized her artistic inclination and provided her with art supplies and dedicated space for creative expression. Engaging in painting and other artistic endeavors, Maria rediscovered her passion and sense of purpose. Her artworks were proudly displayed within the community, and she began teaching art classes to her fellow residents. Through the Montessori approach, Maria's life was transformed, and her talent and enthusiasm brought joy and inspiration to those around her.

Henry's Joy of Gardening:

Henry, a retired gardener, had moved to an assisted living facility where he deeply missed tending to his beloved plants and flowers. Recognizing his passion for gardening, the caregivers incorporated a garden space within the community, providing Henry with the opportunity to continue his gardening pursuits. With adaptive tools and guidance, Henry began nurturing a variety of plants and flowers. His involvement in gardening not only brought him immense joy but also fostered connections with other gardening enthusiasts within the community. Henry's green thumb and passion for gardening revitalized his spirit and showcased the positive impact of the Montessori approach in promoting engagement, purpose, and social connections.

The real-life examples of successful implementation of Montessori for seniors highlight the transformative power of this approach in enhancing well-being and improving the quality of life for older adults. From promoting independence and personal growth to rediscovering passions and fostering social connections, the Montessori philosophy has demonstrated its ability to inspire positive outcomes. These stories serve as a testament to the effectiveness of the Montessori approach in senior care, inspiring caregivers and senior care professionals to embrace and implement its principles, ultimately benefiting the lives of seniors under their care.

www.ingramcontent.com/pod-product-compliance
Lightning Source LLC
Chambersburg PA
CBHW030504220526
45464CB00006B/2652